Meditation

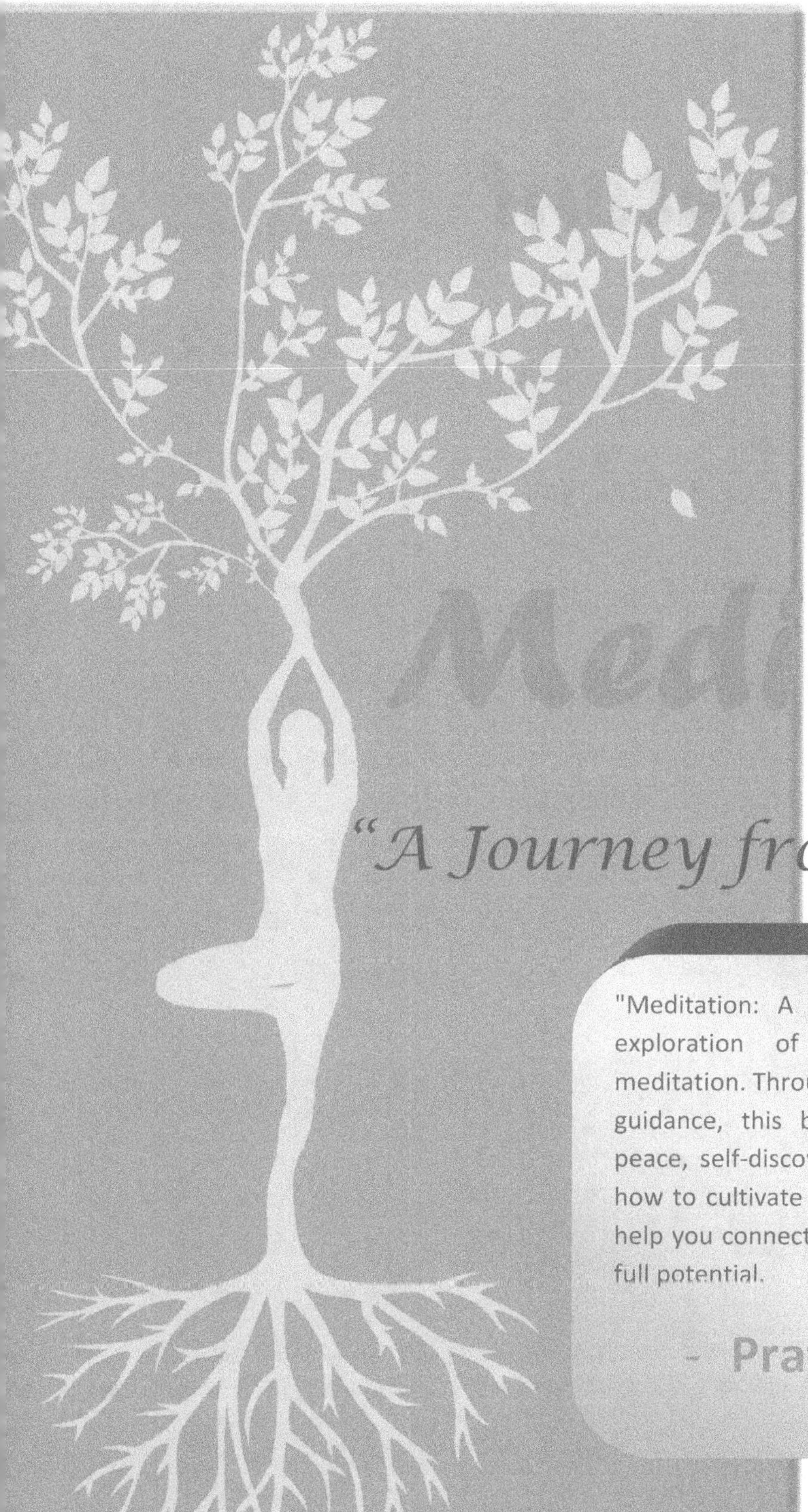

"A Journey from Self to Self"

"Meditation: A Journey from Self to Self" is an exploration of the transformative power of meditation. Through personal anecdotes and practical guidance, this book offers a path towards inner peace, self-discovery, and spiritual growth. Discover how to cultivate a daily meditation practice that will help you connect with your true self and unlock your full potential.

- Pratyaksha Chaurasia

Content

Acknowledgement

Acknowledgement

I am feeling honored in thanking my readers, my family and my husband for motivating me to write this book which have power to change people and their thoughts.

I also owe the credit for the content to various websites which have given me sufficient information to write this book. Dear reader! This book contains various methods of meditation which can guide you to improve yourself and make a better person.

Mindfulness Meditation

Mindfulness meditation is a type of meditation that has gained popularity in recent years, as more and more people seek ways to manage stress, anxiety, and other mental health concerns. It involves paying attention to the present moment, without judgment or distraction, and can be practiced in a variety of settings.

The goal of mindfulness meditation is to increase awareness and clarity of the mind, and to cultivate a sense of peace and well-being. It has been shown to have numerous benefits for mental and physical health, including reducing stress, improving sleep, and enhancing overall well-being.

Here is a complete guide to mindfulness meditation, including its benefits, techniques, and how to get started:

Benefits of Mindfulness Meditation

Research has shown that mindfulness meditation can have numerous benefits for mental and physical health, including:

1. **Reducing stress and anxiety:** Mindfulness meditation can help to reduce stress and anxiety by increasing awareness of thoughts and feelings, and developing the ability to observe them without judgment.

2. *Improving mood:* Practicing mindfulness meditation has been shown to improve mood and reduce symptoms of depression, by increasing awareness of negative thought patterns and learning to disengage from them.

3. *Enhancing focus and concentration:* Mindfulness meditation can help to improve focus and concentration by training the mind to stay present and avoid distraction.

4. *Increasing self-awareness:* Mindfulness meditation can help to increase self-awareness by increasing awareness of thoughts, feelings, and physical sensations in the body.

5. *Improving sleep:* Practicing mindfulness meditation has been shown to improve sleep quality and reduce insomnia, by promoting relaxation and reducing stress.

Technique for Mindfulness Meditation

If you're interested in practicing mindfulness meditation, here are some tips to help you get started:

1. **_Find a comfortable place:_** _For meditation your place need to be comfortable because you can easily get distracted if your body is not in its comfort zone._

2. **_Sit-down on an asana (mat):_** _If you are going under meditation, it is important for you to always sit on an asana because if you will sit on land directly, the land will absorb too much positive from total positive energy that you will make during meditation._

3. **_Close your eyes and calm yourself:_** _After sitting on an asana you need to close your eyes to cut your connection from outer world. Then let yourself calm._
   To calm yourself, you can long inhale and exhale for 2-3 times. Then bring artificial smile on your face. This is not mandatory but, will help you to calm yourself easily.

4. **_Observe your thoughts as a witness:_** _Since thoughts come in our brain non-stop, we cannot stop them from coming. In Mindfulness Meditation you use these thoughts to meditate yourself. I this process you only need to let your thoughts come and go. Either those are good or bad, you need to accept them as it is. You will only observe them as a witness. You will not disturb them. There is difference between thinking and meditation. You will meditate not think._

5. ***Leave yourself free:*** *Slowly-slowly you will go deep in meditation. You do not need to make any effort to do that. It will happen automatically. You only need to leave yourself free. Neither you will do anything nor think. You will free yourself.*

6. ***Be aware of your surroundings:*** *You cannot open your eyes immediately if you are sleeping or meditating. Before opening your eyes, you need to become aware of place where you are. Observe things around yourself then slowly-slowly open your eyes.*

7. ***Make a routine of 15-20 minute meditation:*** *Meditation is not thing to do anytime anywhere. To get better result one should set a fix time for meditation daily of 15-20 minutes. Once you get habitual, you can increase time of meditation.*

Transcendental Meditation

Transcendental meditation (TM) is a type of meditation that was developed in the mid-1950s by **Maharishi Mahesh Yogi**. It is a simple, natural, and effortless technique that involves the use of a mantra, or a sound or word, to help the mind achieve a state of deep relaxation and transcendence.

The technique of TM involves sitting comfortably with your eyes closed, and silently repeating a mantra, which is a sound or word that has no specific meaning. The mantra is chosen by a certified TM teacher, and is meant to be used as a vehicle to transcend or go beyond the surface level of the mind.

The practice of TM is typically done for 20 minutes twice a day, once in the morning and once in the evening. The technique is easy to learn and can be practiced by anyone, regardless of age or background.

Benefits of Transcendental Meditation

TM has been shown to have numerous benefits for mental and physical health, including:

1. **Reducing stress and anxiety:** TM has been shown to reduce stress and anxiety by promoting a state of deep relaxation and reducing the levels of stress hormones in the body.

2. **Improving mood:** TM has been shown to improve mood and reduce symptoms of depression, by promoting relaxation and reducing negative thought patterns.

3. **Enhancing focus and concentration:** TM has been shown to improve focus and concentration by promoting a state of deep relaxation and reducing distraction.

4. **Reducing blood pressure:** TM has been shown to reduce blood pressure and improve cardiovascular health.

5. **Improving sleep:** TM has been shown to improve sleep quality and reduce insomnia, by promoting relaxation and reducing stress.

6. **Increasing self-awareness:** TM has been shown to increase self-awareness and promote a sense of inner calm and well-being.

Technique for Transcendental Meditation

If you're interested in learning TM, here are some steps to get started:

1. **Find a certified TM teacher:** TM can only be learned from a certified TM teacher. You can find a teacher in your area by visiting the official TM website.

2. **Attend an introductory talk:** TM teachers offer introductory talks that explain the benefits and techniques of TM. Attend one of these talks to learn more and decide if TM is right for you.

3. **Schedule a course of instruction:** TM is typically learned in a course of instruction that includes personal instruction and follow-up support. The course may last several days or weeks, and may involve group instruction or one-on-one instruction.

4. **Practice regularly:** Once you have learned TM, it's important to practice regularly to experience the full benefits of the technique. Aim to practice twice a day, once in the morning and once in the evening.

Dear reader! This is not important to practice all type of methods I have mentioned in this book. If you do not waste any more money to learn meditation, you can avoid this chapter. For good result you can choose anyone or more meditation of your choice and practice it daily.

Loving-kindness or Metta or Maitri Meditation

Loving-kindness meditation is a type of meditation that focuses on cultivating feelings of love, kindness, and compassion towards oneself and others. The compassion and universal loving-kindness concept of Metta is discussed in the Metta Sutta of Buddhism, and is also found in the ancient and medieval texts of Hinduism and Jainism as Metta or Maitri.

The practice of Loving-kindness meditation involves sitting comfortably in a quiet place and bringing to mind a person or group of people that you wish to send love and kindness to. This can be you, a loved one, a friend, an acquaintance, a stranger, or even an enemy. You then repeat positive phrases or intentions towards that person, such as "May you be happy, healthy, and peaceful" or "May you be free from suffering and pain."

The practice of Loving-kindness meditation typically involves four stages or levels:

1. **Loving-kindness towards oneself:** The first stage involves directing loving-kindness towards oneself. This involves repeating phrases such as "May I be happy, healthy, and peaceful" or "May I be free from suffering and pain."

2. **Loving-kindness towards a loved one:** The second stage involves directing loving-kindness towards someone you love, such as a family member, a friend, or a partner. This involves repeating phrases such as "May you be

happy, healthy, and peaceful" or "May you be free from suffering and pain."

3. **Loving-kindness towards an acquaintance:** The third stage involves directing loving-kindness towards someone you know but may not have a close relationship with, such as a colleague, neighbor, or acquaintance.

4. **Loving-kindness towards all beings:** The fourth stage involves directing loving-kindness towards all beings, including those you may not know or those who have harmed you. This involves repeating phrases such as "May all beings be happy, healthy, and peaceful" or "May all beings be free from suffering and pain."

Benefits of Loving-kindness meditation

Loving-kindness meditation has been shown to have numerous benefits for mental and physical health, including:

1. **Reducing stress and anxiety:** Loving-kindness meditation has been shown to reduce stress and anxiety by promoting positive emotions and reducing negative thought patterns.

2. **_Improving mood:_** _Loving-kindness meditation has been shown to improve mood and reduce symptoms of depression, by promoting positive emotions and reducing negative thought patterns._

3. **_Enhancing empathy and compassion:_** _Loving-kindness meditation has been shown to enhance empathy and compassion towards oneself and others, by cultivating positive emotions and reducing negative thought patterns._

4. **_Improving relationships:_** _Loving-kindness meditation has been shown to improve relationships by promoting positive emotions and reducing negative thought patterns towards oneself and others._

5. **_Reducing inflammation:_** _Loving-kindness meditation has been shown to reduce inflammation in the body, which can have positive effects on physical health._

Technique of Loving-kindness meditation

If you're interested in trying Loving-kindness meditation, here are some steps to get started:

1. **Find a quiet and comfortable place:** Choose a quiet and comfortable place where you can sit comfortably without being disturbed.

2. **Sit-down on an asana (mat):** If you are going under meditation, it is important for you to always sit on an asana because if you will sit on land directly, the land will absorb too much positive from total positive energy that you will make during meditation.

3. **Close your eyes and calm yourself:** After sitting on an asana you need to close your eyes to cut your connection from outer world. Then let yourself calm.
   To calm yourself, you can long inhale and exhale for 2-3 times. Then bring artificial smile on your face. This is not mandatory but, will help you to calm yourself easily.

4. **Choose a positive phrase or intention:** Choose a positive phrase or intention that resonates with you, such as "May I be happy, healthy, and peaceful" or "May all beings be free from suffering and pain."

5. **Repeat the phrase or intention:** Repeat the phrase or intention in your mind or out loud, directing it towards yourself, a loved one, an acquaintance, or all beings.

8. **Leave yourself free:** After sometime, you will stop repeating phrase and observe all sensations coming from your body. You do not need to make any effort to do that, just a little bit attention is sufficient.
Slowly-slowly you will reach deep in meditation. Now you need to leave yourself. This will calm your inner soul.

9. **Be aware of your surroundings:** You cannot open your eyes immediately if you are sleeping or meditating. Before opening your eyes, you need to become aware of place where you are. Observe things around yourself then slowly-slowly open your eyes.

6. **Practice regularly:** Aim to practice Loving-kindness meditation regularly, for at least 10-15 minutes a day, to experience the full benefits of the technique. Once you become habitual, you can increase the time.

Dear reader! If you are Hindu so you can recite –

सर्वे भवन्तु सुखनिः ।

सर्वे सन्तु निरामयाः ।

सर्वे भद्राणि पश्यन्तु ।

मा कश्चित् दुःख भाग्भवेत् ॥

ॐ शान्तिः शान्तिः शान्तिः॥

This is quite popular in Hindus and some other related religions.

Method - 4

Body scan Meditation

Body scan meditation is a technique that involves systematically focusing on different parts of the body, from head to toe, and bringing awareness to sensations and feelings in each area. This type of meditation is often used for stress reduction, relaxation, and physical and emotional healing.

The practice of body scan meditation typically involves lying down in a comfortable position and starting with a few deep breaths to help relax the body and mind. The meditator then begins to focus on each part of the body, starting at the head and moving down to the toes. The meditator may focus on each body part for a few seconds or several minutes, paying attention to any sensations, such as tension, warmth, or tingling, and acknowledging any emotions or thoughts that arise.

During the practice of body scan meditation, it's important to approach each body part with a sense of curiosity and openness, without judgment or attachment to any sensations or feelings that arise. The goal is to simply observe and become aware of the present moment experience in each area of the body.

Benefits of Body Scan Meditation

Body scan meditation has been shown to have numerous benefits for mental and physical health, including:

1. **Reducing stress and anxiety:** Body scan meditation has been shown to reduce stress and anxiety by promoting relaxation and decreasing negative thought patterns.

2. **Improving sleep:** Body scan meditation has been shown to improve sleep quality and reduce insomnia by promoting relaxation and reducing physical tension.

3. **Increasing body awareness:** Body scan meditation can help increase awareness of physical sensations and feelings in the body, which can help individuals better understand and respond to their own physical and emotional needs.

4. **Enhancing mindfulness:** Body scan meditation can enhance mindfulness by helping individuals focus their attention on the present moment and develop a non-judgmental awareness of their thoughts, feelings, and sensations.

Technique for Body Scan Meditation

If you're interested in trying body scan meditation, here are some steps to get started:

1. **Find a quiet and comfortable place:** Choose a quiet place where you can sit or lie down comfortably without being disturbed.

2. **Sit-down or lie down on an asana (mat):** If you are going under meditation, it is important for you to always use an asana because if you will sit or lie on land directly, the land will absorb too much positive energy from total positive energy that you will make during meditation.

3. **Close your eyes and relax the body:** Now close your eyes and start with a few deep breaths to help relax the body and mind.

4. **Focus on each body part:** Begin to focus on each part of the body, starting at the head and moving down to the toes, or starting at the toes and moving down to the head. Bring awareness to any sensations or feelings in each area.

5. **Be aware of your surroundings:** Before opening your eyes, you need to become aware of place where you are.

Observe things around yourself then sit down if you are lying. Then slowly-slowly open your eyes.

6. **Practice regularly:** *Aim to practice body scan meditation regularly, for at least 10-15 minutes a day. Once you start feeling habitual, you can increase time.*

Overall, body scan meditation is a simple and effective technique for increasing body awareness, reducing stress and anxiety, and promoting relaxation and mindfulness. By bringing awareness to the present moment experience in each part of the body, individuals can develop a deeper understanding and connection to their physical and emotional needs, leading to greater well-being and resilience.

Breath awareness Meditation

Breath awareness meditation is a technique that involves focusing on the breath as a way to bring attention to the present moment. This type of meditation is often used for stress reduction, relaxation, and improving concentration.

The practice of breath awareness meditation typically involves finding a quiet and comfortable place to sit or lie down, closing the eyes, and bringing attention to the sensation of the breath as it moves in and out of the body. The meditator may focus on the sensation of the breath at the nose or the rise and fall of the chest or abdomen.

During the practice of breath awareness meditation, the goal is to maintain focus on the breath while allowing other thoughts and sensations to come and go without judgment or attachment. When the mind inevitably wanders, the meditator simply brings their attention back to the breath and the present moment.

Benefits of Breath Awareness Meditation

Breath awareness meditation has been shown to have numerous benefits for mental and physical health, including:

1. **Reducing stress and anxiety:** Breath awareness meditation has been shown to reduce stress and anxiety

by promoting relaxation and decreasing negative thought patterns.

2. ***Improving focus and concentration:*** *Breath awareness meditation can improve focus and concentration by training the mind to stay present and aware of the breath.*

3. ***Increasing self-awareness:*** *Breath awareness meditation can increase self-awareness by helping individuals observe their thoughts and emotions without judgment, which can lead to greater understanding and acceptance of oneself.*

4. ***Enhancing mindfulness:*** *Breath awareness meditation can enhance mindfulness by helping individuals develop a non-judgmental awareness of their thoughts, feelings, and sensations.*

Technique for Breath Awareness Meditation

If you're interested in trying breath awareness meditation, here are some steps to get started:

1. ***Find a quiet and comfortable place:*** *Choose a quiet and comfortable place where you can sit or lie down comfortably without being disturbed.*

2. ***Sit-down on an asana (mat):*** *If you are going under meditation, it is important for you to always sit on an asana because if you will sit on land directly, the land will absorb too much positive from total positive energy that you will make during meditation.*

3. ***Close your eyes and relax the body:*** *Close your eyes then take a few deep breaths to help relax the body and mind. You can also make an artificial smile to feel more relaxed.*

4. ***Focus on the breath:*** *Bring attention to the sensation of the breath as it moves in and out of the body. You don't need to work hard with your breath or change the rhythm of inhale and exhale. You only need to pay attention to the original rhythm of your breath.*

5. **Leave yourself free:** *Slowly-slowly you will go deep in meditation. You do not need to make any effort to do that. It will happen automatically. You only need to leave yourself free. Neither you will do anything nor think. You will free yourself.*

6. **Be aware of your surroundings:** *You cannot open your eyes immediately if you are sleeping or meditating. Before opening your eyes, you need to become aware of place where you are. Observe things around yourself then slowly-slowly open your eyes.*

7. **Practice regularly:** *Aim to practice breath awareness meditation regularly, for at least 10-15 minutes a day, to experience the full benefits of the technique. You can increase time once you starts feeling habitual.*

Overall, breath awareness meditation is a simple and effective technique for increasing mindfulness, reducing stress and anxiety, and improving focus and concentration. By bringing attention to the present moment experience of the breath, individuals can develop greater awareness of their thoughts and emotions, leading to greater well-being and resilience.

Visualization Meditation

Visualization meditation, also known as guided imagery or creative visualization, is a type of meditation that involves using mental imagery to create a desired outcome or experience. This type of meditation is often used for stress reduction, relaxation, and personal growth.

The practice of visualization meditation typically involves finding a quiet and comfortable place to sit or lie down, closing the eyes, and using mental imagery to create a desired experience. The meditator may imagine themselves in a peaceful place, such as a beach or forest, or visualize themselves achieving a goal, such as giving a successful presentation or completing a challenging task.

During the practice of visualization meditation, the meditator focuses on the details of the imagined experience, using all of their senses to create a vivid mental picture. By doing so, the meditator creates a mental state that is conducive to achieving the desired outcome or experience.

Benefits of Visualization Meditation

Visualization meditation has been shown to have numerous benefits for mental and physical health, including:

1. **Reducing stress and anxiety:** *Visualization meditation can reduce stress and anxiety by promoting relaxation and creating a positive mental state.*

2. **Improving self-confidence:** *Visualization meditation can improve self-confidence by creating a mental picture of success and achievement.*

3. **Enhancing performance:** *Visualization meditation can enhance performance by mentally rehearsing a task or situation before it occurs.*

4. **Promoting healing:** *Visualization meditation can promote healing by creating a mental picture of physical and emotional well-being.*

Technique for Visualization Meditation

If you're interested in trying visualization meditation, here are some steps to get started:

1. *Find a quiet and comfortable place:* Choose a quiet and comfortable place where you can sit or lie down comfortably without being disturbed.

2. *Sit-down on an asana (mat):* If you are going under meditation, it is important for you to always sit on an asana because if you will sit on land directly, the land will absorb too much positive from total positive energy that you will make during meditation.

3. *Close your eyes and calm yourself:* After sitting on an asana you need to close your eyes to cut your connection from outer world. Then let yourself calm.
   To calm yourself, you can long inhale and exhale for 2-3 times. Then bring artificial smile on your face. This is not mandatory but, will help you to calm yourself easily.

4. *Choose a visualization:* Choose a visualization that resonates with you, such as a peaceful place or achieving a goal.

5. *Create a mental picture:* Use all of your senses to create a vivid mental picture of the chosen visualization.

6. ***Leave yourself free:*** *Slowly-slowly you will go deep in meditation. You do not need to make any effort to do that. It will happen automatically. You only need to leave yourself free. Neither you will do anything nor think. You will free yourself.*

7. ***Be aware of your surroundings:*** *You cannot open your eyes immediately if you are sleeping or meditating. Before opening your eyes, you need to become aware of place where you are. Observe things around yourself then slowly-slowly open your eyes.*

8. ***Practice regularly:*** *Aim to practice visualization meditation regularly, for at least 10-15 minutes a day, to experience the full benefits of the technique.*

Overall, visualization meditation is a powerful technique for promoting relaxation, reducing stress and anxiety, and achieving personal growth. By creating a positive mental state and visualizing desired outcomes and experiences, individuals can enhance their performance, improve their well-being, and achieve greater success in their lives.

Chakra Meditation

Chakra meditation is a type of meditation that focuses on the seven energy centers, or chakras, located along the spine. These energy centers are believed to correspond to different physical, emotional, and spiritual aspects of the body.

The practice of chakra meditation typically involves finding a quiet and comfortable place to sit or lie down, closing the eyes, and bringing awareness to each of the chakras in turn. The meditator may use visualization, chanting, or breathwork to activate and balance each chakra.

The seven chakras are:

1. **Root Chakra (Muladhara):** Located at the base of the spine, this chakra is associated with grounding, stability, and security.

2. **Sacral Chakra (Svadhisthana):** Located in the lower abdomen, this chakra is associated with creativity, sexuality, and emotional balance.

3. **Solar Plexus Chakra (Manipura):** Located in the upper abdomen, this chakra is associated with personal power, self-esteem, and confidence.

4. *Heart Chakra (Anahata):* Located in the center of the chest, this chakra is associated with love, compassion, and connection.

5. *Throat Chakra (Vishuddha):* Located in the throat, this chakra is associated with communication, self-expression, and authenticity.

6. *Third Eye Chakra (Ajna):* Located in the forehead, this chakra is associated with intuition, clarity, and spiritual insight.

7. *Crown Chakra (Sahasrara):* Located at the top of the head, this chakra is associated with spiritual connection, enlightenment, and unity.

Benefits of Chakra Meditation

Chakra meditation has been shown to have numerous benefits for mental and physical health, including:

1. **Balancing the chakras:** Chakra meditation can balance the energy flow in the body and promote overall well-being.

2. **Reducing stress and anxiety:** Chakra meditation can reduce stress and anxiety by promoting relaxation and balancing the emotions.

3. **Enhancing spiritual growth:** Chakra meditation can enhance spiritual growth by promoting awareness and connection with the divine.

4. **Improving physical health:** Chakra meditation can improve physical health by promoting healing and balancing the body's systems.

Technique for Chakra Meditation

If you're interested in trying chakra meditation, here are some steps to get started:

1. **Find a quiet and comfortable place:** Choose a quiet and comfortable place where you can sit or lie down comfortably without being disturbed.

2. **Sit-down on an asana (mat):** If you are going under meditation, it is important for you to always sit on an asana because if you will sit on land directly, the land will absorb too much positive from total positive energy that you will make during meditation.

3. **Close your eyes and calm yourself:** After sitting on an asana you need to close your eyes to cut your connection from outer world. Then let yourself calm.
To calm yourself, you can long inhale and exhale for 2-3 times. Then bring artificial smile on your face. This is not mandatory but, will help you to calm yourself easily.

4. **Bring awareness to each chakra:** Focus on each chakra from Root Chakra to Crown Chakra in turn, using visualization, chanting, or breath-work to activate and balance the energy.

5. **Leave yourself free:** After reaching Crown Chakra, you will observe sensations of your body. Then slowly-slowly leave yourself free. Neither you will do anything nor think. You will free yourself.

6. **Be aware of your surroundings:** *Before opening your eyes, you need to become aware of place where you are. Observe things around yourself then slowly-slowly open your eyes.*

7. **Practice regularly:** *Aim to practice chakra meditation regularly, for at least 10-15 minutes a day, to experience the full benefits of the technique.*

Overall, chakra meditation is a powerful technique for promoting balance, relaxation, and spiritual growth. By bringing awareness to the energy centers in the body and using visualization and other techniques to balance and activate them, individuals can promote overall well-being and enhance their connection with the divine.

Method - 8

Vipassana Meditation

Vipassana meditation is a type of meditation that originated in ancient India and has been practiced for over 2,500 years. The word "vipassana" means insight or clear seeing, and the practice involves cultivating a deep awareness and understanding of one's thoughts, emotions, and physical sensations.

The practice of Vipassana meditation typically involves finding a quiet and comfortable place to sit or lie down, closing the eyes, and focusing on the breath or physical sensations in the body. The meditator observes these sensations with detachment, allowing them to arise and pass away without judgment or attachment.

During the practice of Vipassana meditation, the goal is to develop a deep awareness of one's inner experience, including thoughts, emotions, and physical sensations. By doing so, individuals can develop insight into the nature of their own mind and the causes of suffering, and ultimately achieve a state of inner peace and happiness.

Benefits of Vipassana Meditation

Vipassana meditation has been shown to have numerous benefits for mental and physical health, including:

1. **Reducing stress and anxiety:** Vipassana meditation can reduce stress and anxiety by promoting relaxation and cultivating a deep sense of inner peace.

2. **Improving emotional regulation:** Vipassana meditation can improve emotional regulation by helping individuals develop awareness and detachment from their thoughts and emotions.

3. **Enhancing focus and concentration:** Vipassana meditation can enhance focus and concentration by training the mind to stay present and focused on the present moment.

4. **Promoting self-awareness:** Vipassana meditation can promote self-awareness by cultivating a deep understanding of one's own thoughts, emotions, and physical sensations.

Technique for Vipassana Meditation

If you're interested in trying Vipassana meditation, here are some steps to get started:

1. ***Find a quiet and comfortable place:*** *Choose a quiet and comfortable place where you can sit or lie down comfortably without being disturbed.*

2. ***Sit-down on an asana (mat):*** *If you are going under meditation, it is important for you to always sit on an asana because if you will sit on land directly, the land will absorb too much positive from total positive energy that you will make during meditation.*

3. ***Close your eyes and calm yourself:*** *After sitting on an asana you need to close your eyes to cut your connection from outer world. Then let yourself calm.*
To calm yourself, you can long inhale and exhale for 2-3 times. Then bring artificial smile on your face. This is not mandatory but, will help you to calm yourself easily.

4. ***Focus on the breath or physical sensations:*** *Focus on the breath or physical sensations in the body, observing them with detachment.*

5. ***Observe thoughts and emotions:*** *When thoughts or emotions arise, observe them with detachment and let them pass without judgment or attachment.*

6. ***Leave yourself free:*** *Slowly-slowly you will go deep in meditation. You do not need to make any effort to do that. It will happen automatically. You only need to leave yourself free. Neither you will do anything nor think. You will free yourself.*

7. ***Be aware of your surroundings:*** *You cannot open your eyes immediately if you are sleeping or meditating. Before opening your eyes, you need to become aware of place where you are. Observe things around yourself then sit down if you are lying. Then slowly-slowly open your eyes.*

8. ***Practice regularly:*** *Aim to practice Vipassana meditation regularly, for at least 10-15 minutes a day, to experience the full benefits of the technique.*

Overall, Vipassana meditation is a powerful technique for promoting self-awareness, reducing stress and anxiety, and achieving a state of inner peace and happiness. By cultivating a deep awareness of one's inner experience and learning to observe thoughts and emotions with detachment, individuals can develop insight into the nature of their own mind and achieve a greater sense of well-being.

Zen Meditation

Zen meditation, also known as Zazen, is a type of meditation that originated in ancient China and Japan and is widely practiced in Zen Buddhism. The practice involves sitting in a specific posture and focusing on the breath or a specific object, while maintaining a state of deep relaxation and alertness.

The practice of Zen meditation typically involves finding a quiet and comfortable place to sit, often on a meditation cushion or mat, and assuming a specific posture. The posture involves sitting upright with the legs crossed and the hands placed in the lap or on the knees, with the spine straight and the chin tucked in slightly.

During the practice of Zen meditation, the goal is to maintain a state of deep relaxation and alertness, while focusing on the breath or a specific object. The meditator may use specific techniques, such as counting the breaths or repeating a mantra, to help maintain focus and concentration.

Benefits of Zen Meditation

Zen meditation has been shown to have numerous benefits for mental and physical health, including:

1. **Reducing stress and anxiety:** Zen meditation can reduce stress and anxiety by promoting relaxation and cultivating a sense of inner peace.

2. *Improving focus and concentration:* Zen meditation can improve focus and concentration by training the mind to stay present and focused on the present moment.

3. *Promoting emotional regulation:* Zen meditation can promote emotional regulation by helping individuals develop awareness and detachment from their thoughts and emotions.

4. *Enhancing overall well-being:* Zen meditation can enhance overall well-being by promoting a sense of calm, relaxation, and inner peace.

Technique for Zen Meditation

If you're interested in trying Zen meditation, here are some steps to get started:

1. *Find a quiet and comfortable place:* Choose a quiet and comfortable place where you can sit comfortably without being disturbed.

2. **Sit-down on an asana (mat):** If you are going under meditation, it is important for you to always sit on an asana because if you will sit on land directly, the land will absorb too much positive from total positive energy that you will make during meditation.

3. **Assume a specific posture:** Assume a specific posture, such as the cross-legged sitting posture, with the spine straight and the chin tucked in slightly.

4. **Focus on the breath or a specific object:** Focus on the breath or a specific object, such as a candle flame or a mantra, while maintaining a state of deep relaxation and alertness.

5. **Close your eyes and calm yourself:** After sometime, slowly- slowly close your eyes. And let yourself calm.

6. **Leave yourself free:** Slowly-slowly you will go deep in meditation. You do not need to make any effort to do that. It will happen automatically. You only need to leave yourself free. Neither you will do anything nor think. You will free yourself.

7. **Be aware of your surroundings:** You cannot open your eyes immediately if you are sleeping or meditating.

Before opening your eyes, you need to become aware of place where you are. Observe things around yourself then slowly-slowly open your eyes.

8. **Practice regularly:** *Aim to practice Zen meditation regularly, for at least 10-15 minutes a day, to experience the full benefits of the technique.*

Overall, Zen meditation is a powerful technique for promoting relaxation, focus, and emotional regulation. By cultivating a state of deep relaxation and alertness and focusing on the breath or a specific object, individuals can achieve a greater sense of well-being and inner peace.

Method - 10

Yoga Meditation

Yoga meditation is a form of meditation that is closely associated with the practice of yoga, a physical, mental, and spiritual discipline that originated in ancient India. Yoga meditation involves a combination of physical postures, breathing techniques, and meditation practices, with the aim of achieving a sense of inner peace, balance, and harmony.

The practice of yoga meditation typically involves assuming a series of physical postures, known as asanas, while focusing on the breath and maintaining a state of deep relaxation and awareness. Asanas are typically held for a few minutes at a time, and are designed to stretch and strengthen the body, while also promoting relaxation and focus.

In addition to the physical postures, yoga meditation also involves specific breathing techniques, known as pranayama, which are designed to calm the mind, reduce stress and anxiety, and increase overall vitality and well-being. These breathing techniques involve various patterns of inhaling and exhaling, and are often combined with specific hand gestures, or mudras.

Finally, the practice of yoga meditation also involves various forms of meditation, which can include focused concentration, visualization, or mindfulness practices. These meditation techniques are designed to help individuals develop a deeper sense of awareness, and to cultivate a sense of inner peace and tranquility.

Benefits of Yoga Meditation

The practice of yoga meditation has numerous benefits for mental and physical health, including:

1. **Stress reduction:** The combination of physical postures, breathwork, and meditation can help reduce stress and promote relaxation.

2. **Improved mental clarity:** The practice of yoga meditation can help improve mental clarity and focus by calming the mind and promoting mindfulness.

3. **Increased flexibility and strength:** The physical postures of yoga can improve flexibility and strength, which can lead to better overall physical health.

4. **Better sleep:** The relaxation and mindfulness promoted by yoga meditation can help improve sleep quality and duration.

Technique for Yoga Meditation

If you're interested in trying yoga meditation, here are some steps to get started:

1. **Find a quiet and comfortable space:** Choose a quiet and comfortable space where you can practice yoga meditation without being disturbed.

2. **Choose a comfortable position:** Choose a comfortable position for your body, such as sitting on a cushion or a chair with your back straight.

3. **Focus on the breath:** Begin by focusing on your breath, taking slow, deep breaths in and out through your nose.

4. **Practice physical postures:** Move through a series of physical postures, such as downward dog or warrior pose, to help release tension and promote flexibility.

5. **Practice meditation:** After you've completed the physical postures, move into a seated meditation posture and focus on your breath or a specific object, such as a mantra.

6. **End with relaxation:** End your yoga meditation practice with a few minutes of relaxation, such as lying in savasana (corpse pose), to help integrate the benefits of the practice into your body and mind.

Overall, the practice of yoga meditation can be a powerful tool for promoting relaxation, mindfulness, and overall well-being. By combining physical postures, breathwork, and meditation, individuals can cultivate a greater sense of inner peace and connection to the present moment.

Walking Meditation

Walking meditation is a form of meditation that involves walking slowly and mindfully, while focusing on the present moment and the sensations of the body. It can be practiced outdoors or indoors, in a quiet space or in a public area, and is accessible to people of all ages and fitness levels.

In walking meditation, the goal is to maintain a state of mindfulness and awareness as you walk, focusing on the sensations of the body and the movement of the feet. The practice can be done in silence or with a guided meditation, and can be tailored to meet the needs and preferences of the individual practitioner.

Benefits of Walking Meditation

Walking meditation has numerous benefits for mental and physical health, including:

1. **Stress reduction:** Walking meditation can help reduce stress and promote relaxation by slowing down the mind and focusing on the present moment.

2. **Improved focus and concentration:** Walking meditation can improve focus and concentration by training the mind to stay present and focused on the sensations of the body.

3. **Increased physical activity:** Walking meditation can increase physical activity levels, which can have numerous benefits for overall physical health.

4. **Better sleep:** The relaxation and mindfulness promoted by walking meditation can help improve sleep quality and duration.

Technique for Walking Meditation

If you're interested in trying walking meditation, here are some steps to get started:

1. **Find a quiet space:** Choose a quiet space where you can walk slowly and mindfully without being disturbed.

2. **Stand still and focus:** Stand still for a moment and focus on your breath and the sensations of your body.

3. **Begin walking:** Begin walking slowly, focusing on the sensations of your feet as they touch the ground and the movement of your body.

4. **Stay mindful:** Stay mindful and present as you walk, focusing on your breath and the sensations of your body.

5. **Return to focus:** If your mind wanders, gently return your focus to the sensations of your body and the movement of your feet.

6. **End with reflection:** End your walking meditation practice with a few moments of reflection, focusing on the benefits of the practice and how you can integrate it into your daily life.

Overall, walking meditation can be a powerful tool for promoting relaxation, mindfulness, and overall well-being. By focusing on the present moment and the sensations of the body while walking, individuals can cultivate a greater sense of inner peace and connection to the world around them.

Yoga Nidra

Yoga Nidra is a form of guided meditation that is practiced while lying down in a comfortable and relaxed position, such as savasana (corpse pose). It is a deeply relaxing and rejuvenating practice that can help reduce stress, anxiety, and tension in the body and mind.

Yoga Nidra is often referred to as "yogic sleep" because it induces a state of deep relaxation that is similar to sleep, but with full awareness and consciousness. The practice involves systematically moving the awareness through different parts of the body, while staying in a state of deep relaxation and stillness.

Benefits of Yoga Nidra

Yoga Nidra has numerous benefits for mental and physical health, including:

1. **Stress reduction:** Yoga Nidra can help reduce stress and tension in the body and mind, promoting deep relaxation and calmness.

2. **Improved sleep:** The deep relaxation induced by Yoga Nidra can help improve sleep quality and duration.

3. **Increased awareness:** The practice of Yoga Nidra can help increase awareness and mindfulness, promoting a deeper connection to the present moment.

4. **Reduced anxiety and depression:** Yoga Nidra can help reduce symptoms of anxiety and depression by promoting a sense of calmness and relaxation.

Technique for Yoga Nidra

If you're interested in trying Yoga Nidra, here are some steps to get started:

1. **Find a quiet space:** Choose a quiet and comfortable space where you can lie down and relax without being disturbed.

2. **Get comfortable:** Lie down in savasana (corpse pose) or another comfortable position, with a pillow or blanket if needed.

3. **Follow the guidance:** Listen to a guided Yoga Nidra meditation, either in person or through a recording, and

follow the instructions to relax deeply and move the awareness through different parts of the body.

During Yoga Nidra, the practitioner lies down in a comfortable position and follows a guided meditation that takes them through various stages of relaxation. The practice begins with a body scan, where the practitioner focuses on each part of the body, releasing tension and relaxing muscles.

Next, the practitioner is guided through a visualization or imagery exercise, such as walking through a peaceful forest or floating on a calm ocean. This helps to calm the mind and promote a sense of inner peace.

Finally, the practitioner is guided back to the present moment, becoming aware of their physical surroundings and bringing their awareness back to the present moment. The practice typically lasts for around 20-30 minutes.

4. **Stay present:** Stay present and aware throughout the practice, focusing on the guidance and the sensations in the body.

5. **End with relaxation:** End the practice with a few moments of relaxation and stillness, taking the time to integrate the benefits of the practice into the body and mind.

Overall, Yoga Nidra is considered to be an accessible form of meditation that can be practiced by anyone, regardless of age or physical ability. It is often used as a tool for stress reduction, insomnia, and other health issues related to stress and tension.

The practice of Yoga Nidra can be a powerful tool for promoting relaxation, mindfulness, and overall well-being. By inducing a state of deep relaxation and calmness, individuals can experience a greater sense of inner peace and connection to the present moment.

Japa Meditation

Japa meditation is a type of meditation that involves the repetition of a mantra, a sacred word or phrase, to help focus and quiet the mind. The word "japa" comes from the Sanskrit word "jap," which means "to repeat silently."

The practice of Japa meditation involves repeating the chosen mantra silently to oneself, either by mentally chanting it or whispering it softly. The practitioner may use a mala, a string of beads similar to a rosary, to keep track of the repetitions and help maintain focus.

Benefits of Japa Meditation

Japa meditation has numerous benefits for mental and physical health, including:

1. **Increased focus and concentration:** The repetition of the mantra can help improve focus and concentration by keeping the mind centered on a single point.

2. **Reduced stress and anxiety:** Japa meditation can help reduce stress and anxiety by promoting relaxation and a sense of inner peace.

3. **Spiritual growth:** Japa meditation is often used as a spiritual practice to deepen one's connection to the divine and cultivate a greater sense of inner wisdom and intuition.

4. **Improved mood:** Japa meditation can help improve mood and reduce symptoms of depression by promoting feelings of calm and well-being.

Technique for Japa Meditation

If you're interested in trying Japa meditation, here are some steps to get started:

1. **Choose a mantra:** Choose a mantra that resonates with you, whether it's a sacred word or phrase like "**OM**" or "**Om Namah Shivay!**" etc.

2. **Find a quiet space:** Find a quiet space where you won't be disturbed, and sit comfortably with your eyes closed.

3. **Use a mala:** If you want to chant 108 times, you can use a mala of 108 beads for counting. In that case, hold it in your hand and move one bead at a time with each repetition of the mantra.

4. **Begin repeating the mantra:** Begin repeating the mantra silently to yourself, either mentally or by whispering it softly.

5. **Stay focused:** Stay focused on the mantra and the feeling it creates within you, letting go of any distracting thoughts that may arise.

6. **End with gratitude:** End your Japa meditation practice with a few moments of gratitude and reflection, thanking yourself for taking the time to cultivate inner peace and well-being.

Overall, Japa meditation can be a powerful tool for promoting relaxation, focus, and spiritual growth. By repeating a sacred word or phrase, individuals can cultivate a deeper sense of connection to themselves, to others, and to the world around them.

Method - 14

Trataka Meditation

Trataka meditation, also known as "steady gazing," is a form of meditation that involves focused gazing at a single point or object, such as a candle flame or an image, to help quiet the mind and improve concentration. The practice is said to help awaken intuition, increase awareness, and promote mental clarity.

Benefits of Trataka Meditation

Trataka meditation is said to have numerous benefits for mental and physical health, including:

1. **Improved concentration and focus:** Trataka meditation can help improve concentration and focus by training the mind to stay focused on a single point.

2. **Increased intuition and awareness:** Trataka meditation is believed to help awaken intuition and increase awareness by promoting a state of inner stillness and clarity.

3. **Reduced stress and anxiety:** Trataka meditation can help reduce stress and anxiety by promoting relaxation and calmness.

4. *Improved eyesight:* Trataka meditation is also believed to have a positive effect on eyesight and can help relieve eye strain.

Technique for Trataka Meditation

To practice Trataka meditation, follow these steps:

1. **Find a quiet and comfortable space:** Find a quiet and comfortable space where you won't be disturbed and sit comfortably in a cross-legged position or on a chair with your spine straight.

2. **Choose a focal point:** Choose a focal point, such as a candle flame, a symbol or an image, and place it at eye level, about arm's length away from you.

3. **Gaze at the object:** Begin gazing at the object, focusing your gaze on a single point without blinking for as long as you can. If your eyes become fatigued, you can close them for a few moments before resuming your gaze.

4. **Maintain focus:** Try to maintain your focus on the object, observing its details, its color, and its form, and avoiding any thoughts or distractions that may arise.

5. **End the practice:** When you're ready to end the practice, gently close your eyes and focus on the afterimage of the object in your mind's eye for a few moments before returning to your regular activities.

Overall, Trataka meditation is a simple yet powerful meditation practice that can help improve concentration, promote relaxation, and awaken inner wisdom and intuition.

Kundalini Meditation

Kundalini meditation is a type of meditation that focuses on awakening the dormant Kundalini energy that lies at the base of the spine. This energy is believed to be a powerful source of spiritual energy and consciousness that, when awakened, can bring about transformative experiences and lead to spiritual growth.

Benefits of Kundalini Meditation

Kundalini meditation is said to have numerous benefits for physical, mental, and spiritual health, including:

1. **Increased energy and vitality:** Kundalini meditation is believed to help increase energy and vitality by activating the Kundalini energy, which is said to be a powerful source of spiritual energy.

2. **Improved emotional balance:** Kundalini meditation can help improve emotional balance and reduce stress and anxiety by promoting relaxation and inner peace.

3. **Increased self-awareness and intuition:** Kundalini meditation is believed to help increase self-awareness and

intuition by awakening the inner wisdom and spiritual consciousness.

4. **Spiritual growth and transformation:** Kundalini meditation is said to be a powerful tool for spiritual growth and transformation, leading to greater clarity, insight, and connection to the divine.

Technique for Kundalini Meditation

To practice Kundalini meditation, follow these steps:

1. **Find a quiet and comfortable space:** Find a quiet space where you won't be disturbed and sit comfortably in a cross-legged position or on a chair with your spine straight.

2. **Begin with breathwork:** Close your eyes and begin by taking a few deep breaths, inhaling through your nose and exhaling through your mouth, to help calm your mind and body.

3. **Focus on the Kundalini energy:** Focus your attention on the base of your spine, where the Kundalini energy is said to be located. Visualize the energy as a coiled serpent, waiting to be awakened.

4. **Use mantra and mudra:** Use a mantra, such as "Sat Nam" (meaning "truth is my identity"), and a mudra, such as Gyan mudra (touching the thumb and index finger), to help activate the Kundalini energy.

5. **Allow the energy to flow:** As you repeat the mantra and hold the mudra, allow the Kundalini energy to rise up through your body, passing through each of the seven chakras, or energy centers, along the way.

6. **Experience the energy:** As the Kundalini energy rises, you may experience physical sensations, such as heat, tingling, or vibrations, as well as emotional and spiritual experiences, such as a sense of peace, clarity, or connection to the divine.

7. **End the practice:** When you're ready to end the practice, take a few deep breaths and allow the energy to settle back down to its resting state. You may also want to take some time to journal or reflect on your experience.

Overall, Kundalini meditation is a powerful and transformative meditation practice that can help awaken the inner wisdom and spiritual energy within us, leading to greater physical, mental, and spiritual health and well-being.